The Cure for Anxiety

DISCLAIMER: Always consult with a doctor prior to starting a new treatment.

Table of Contents

What Causes Anxiety? **[4]**

How Does Pathogenic Bacteria Cause Anxiety? **[6]**

The Cure for Anxiety **[8]**

- Step 1: Get Tested **[9]**

- Step 2: Doctor Approved treatment **[12]**

- Step 3: Retest to verify irradiation **[14]**

- Step 4: Clean the remaining toxins from your system **[16]**

Welcome to Real Happiness **[21]**

So What Causes Anxiety?

The primary cause of anxiety is **pathogenic bacteria** in the intestines.

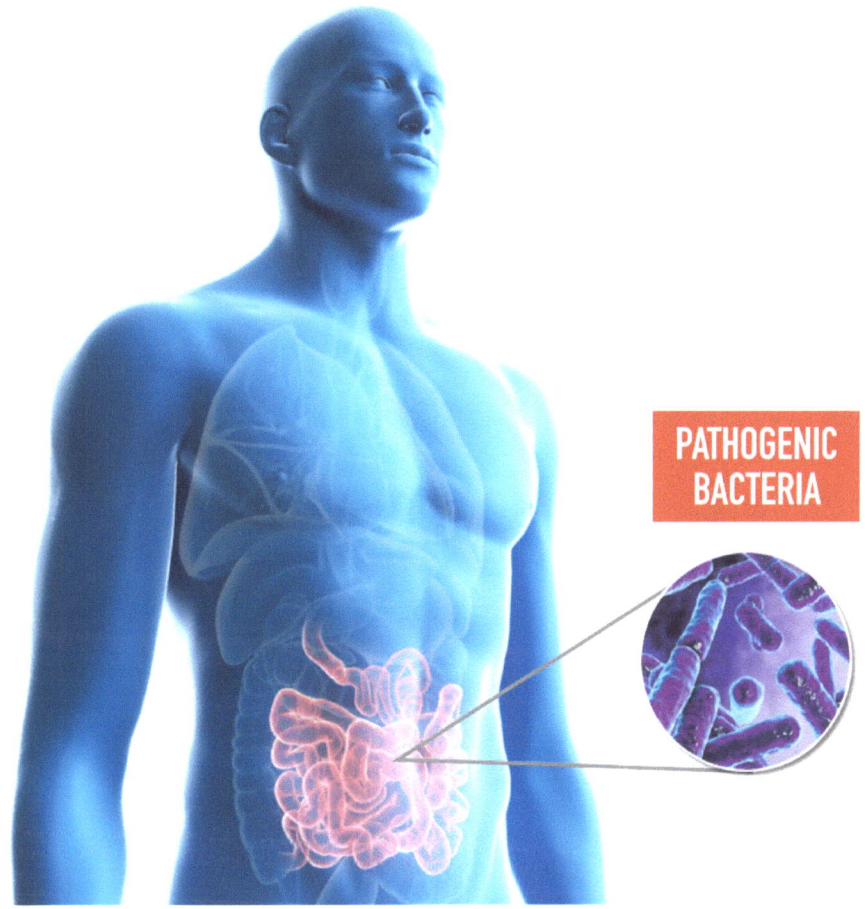

How Does Pathogenic Bacteria Cause Anxiety?

Pathogenic bacteria release toxins that travel to the brain.

When the brain is saturated with toxins, the result is anxiety.

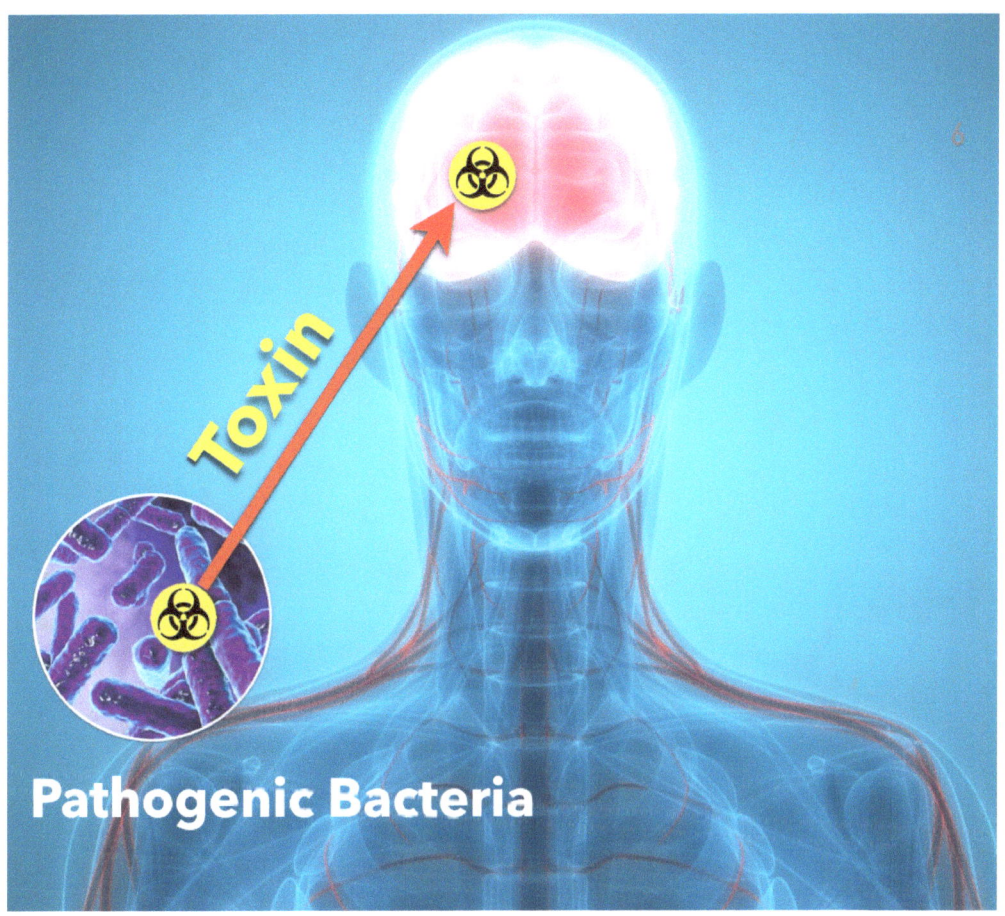

Here is The Cure
for Anxiety

Step 1
Get Tested

The purpose of getting tested is to identify the name of the pathogenic microbes in the intestine. And the best way to do that is to get a **stool test**.

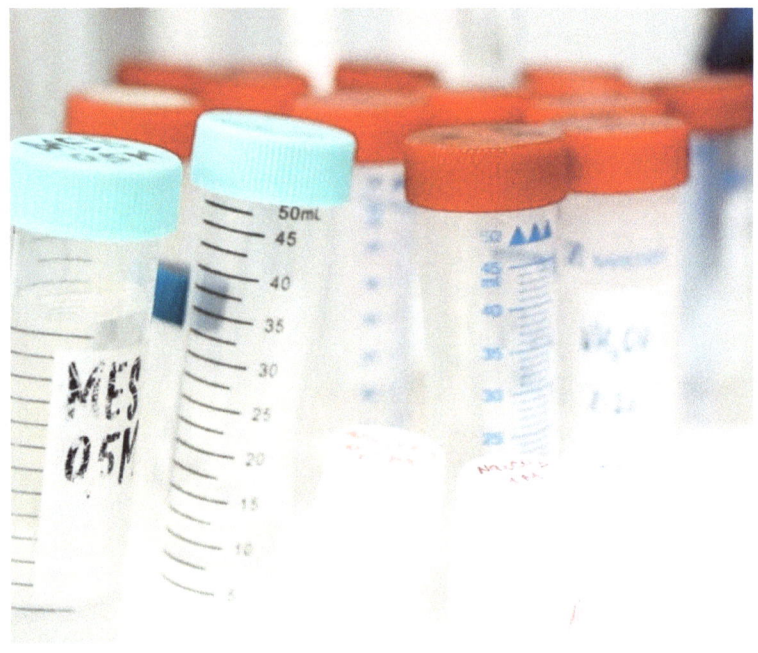

There are 3 stool tests for this purpose (stool is feces, caca):

1. **H. Pylori Stool Test:**
- Helicobacter Pylori is a pathogenic bacteria

2. **Bacterial Culture Stool Test:**
- Shows both pathogenic and beneficial bacteria
- Lab must do an Antimicrobial Susceptibility Test
- PCR tests are the most advanced & accurate
- Don't rely on the lab's definition of whether a bacteria is pathogenic or not, as it can be false. Ask a doctor instead.

3. **Parasite Stool Test:**
- Collected over 3 days

Step 2

Doctor Approved Treatment

When a pathogenic bacteria or microbe is found, your doctor can use the lab's antimicrobial susceptibility test results to determine which treatment will be effective at eradicating the pathogenic bacteria or microbe.

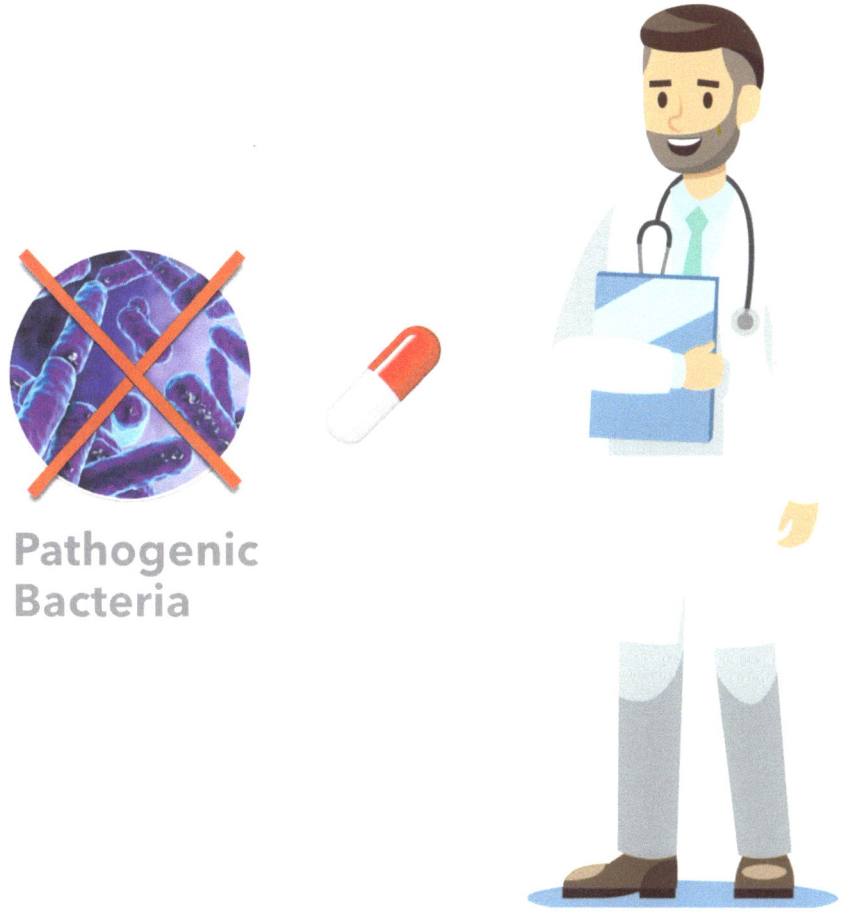

An example of pathogenic bacteria: *Alpha Haemolytic Streptococcus*

Step 3

Re-Test to Verify Eradication

Repeat the test(s) two months after the treatment is finished to verify that the pathogenic bacteria or microbe is eradicated.

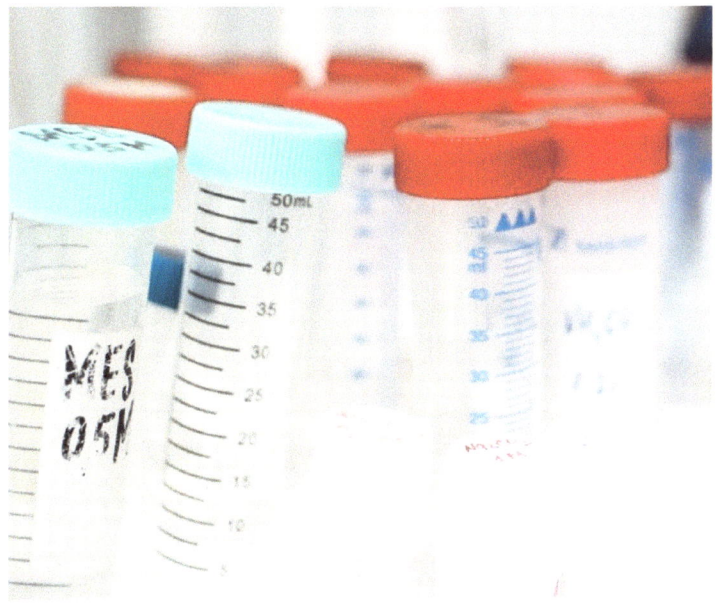

Step 4

Clean the Remaining Toxins

The toxins will remain in your system even after eradicating the pathogenic bacteria.

And in order to undo the disorders that were inflicted on your system, you **must remove the remaining toxins from your body**.

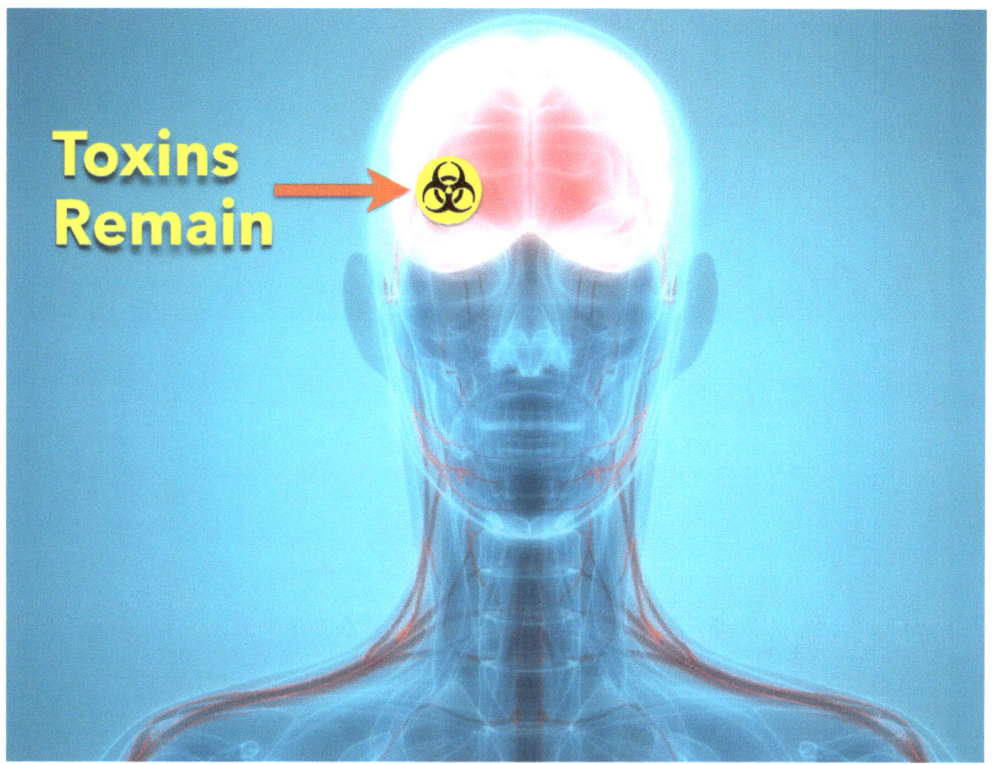

To remove the remaining toxins, you will need the following:

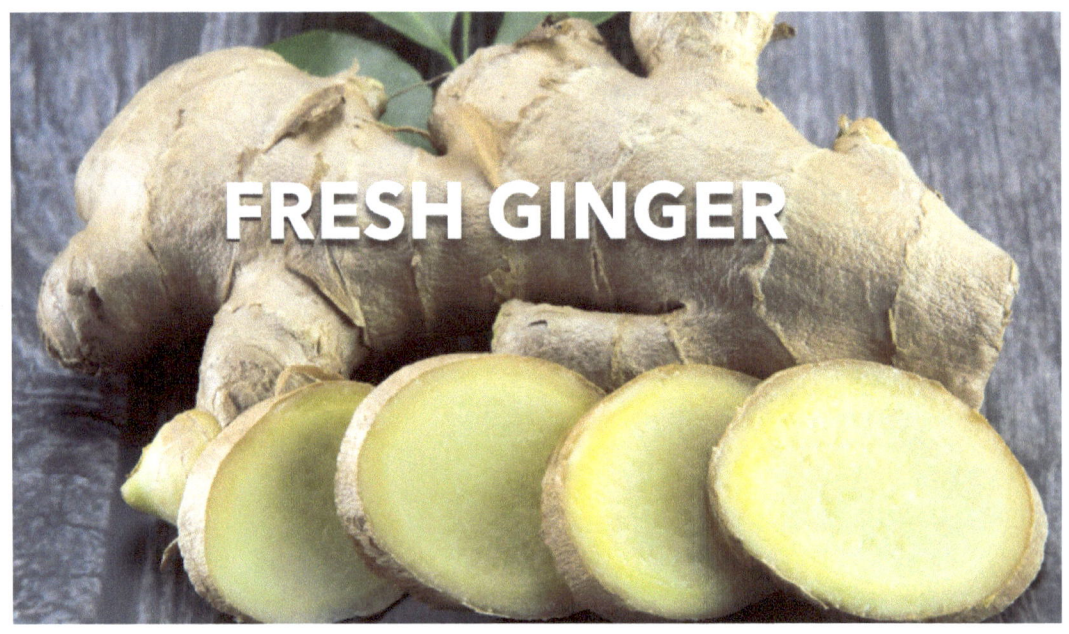

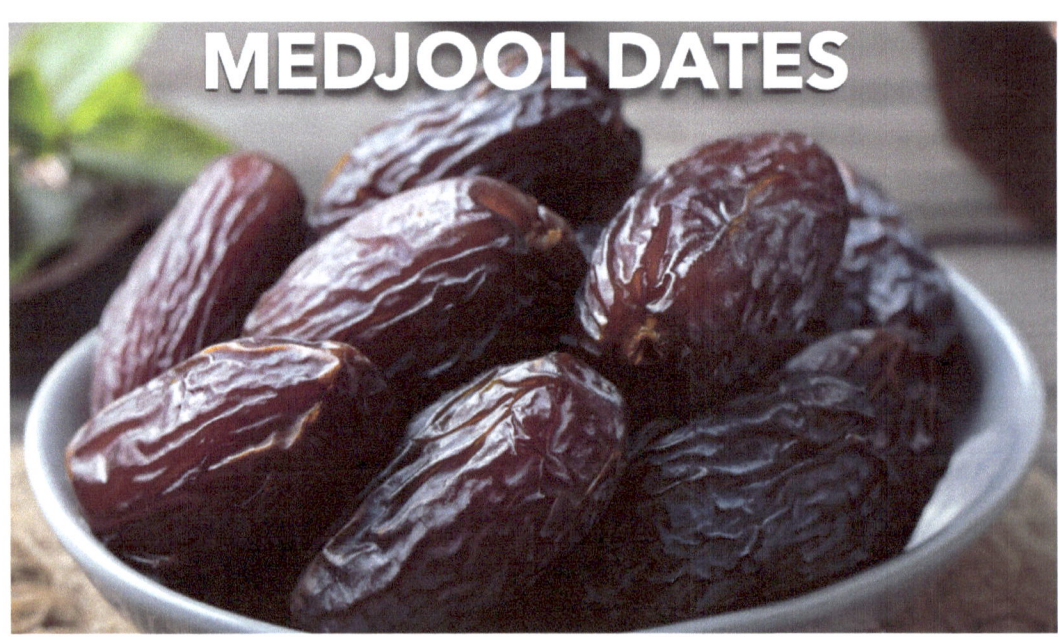

- **Fresh Ginger** disables the leftover toxins for 1 hour
- **Medjool Dates** clean the toxins from your system

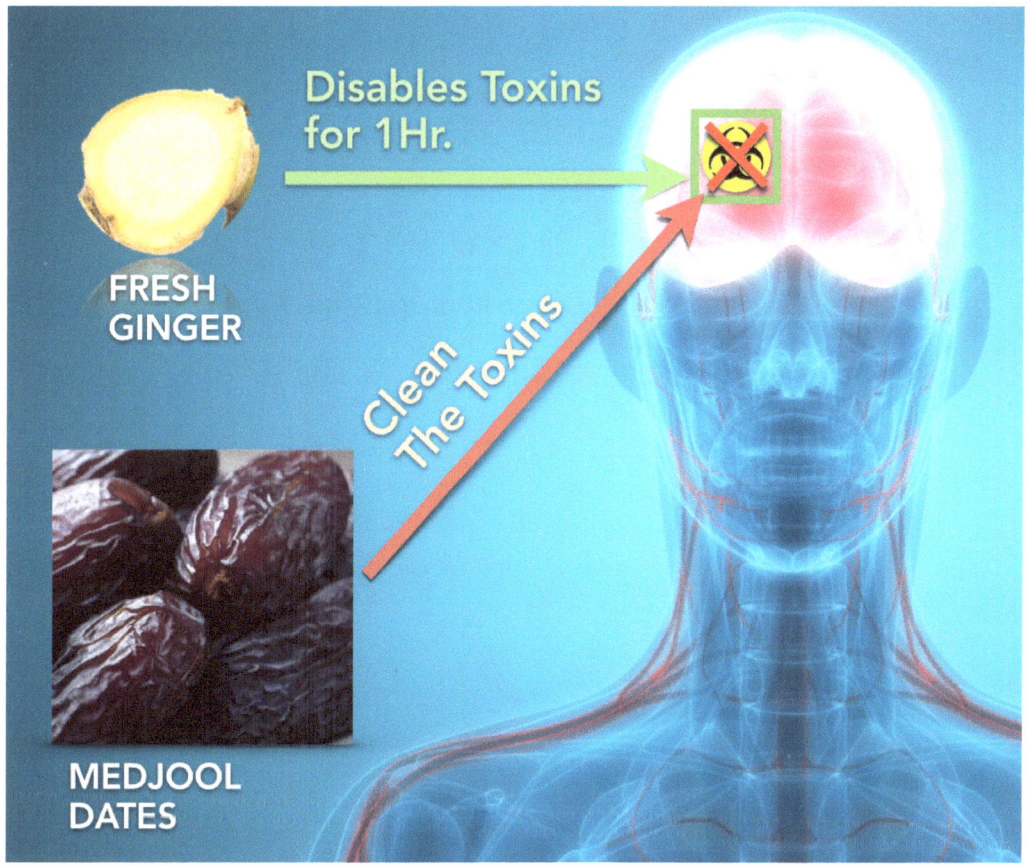

At this point, If you still feel like you have not fully recovered yet, it means either that:

1. There are still some toxins clinging to your system: In this case, you will need some probiotic bacteria that will override the bad toxins that are clinging to your system, and therefore freeing you from their disorders.

OR:

2. There are still some pathogenic microbes in your gut.

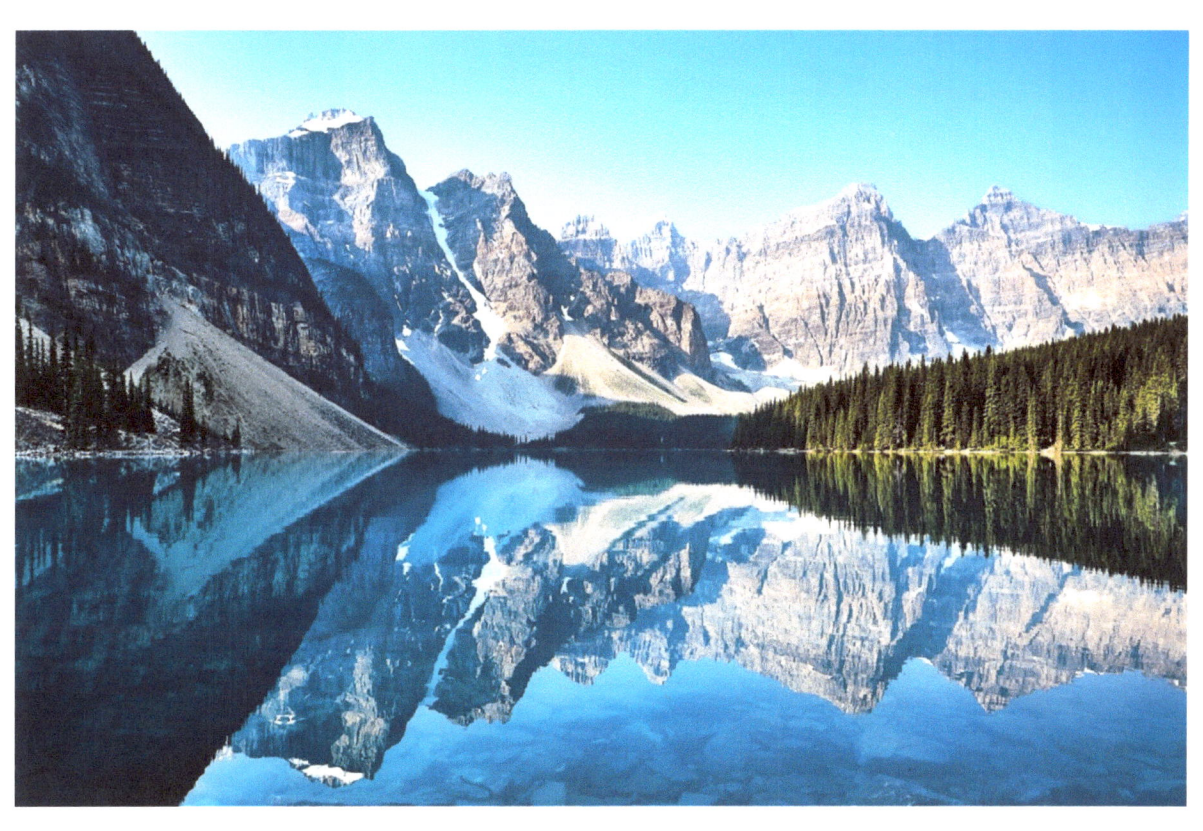

Welcome to Real Happiness

This book is based on real research
conducted on real subjects over 10 years.

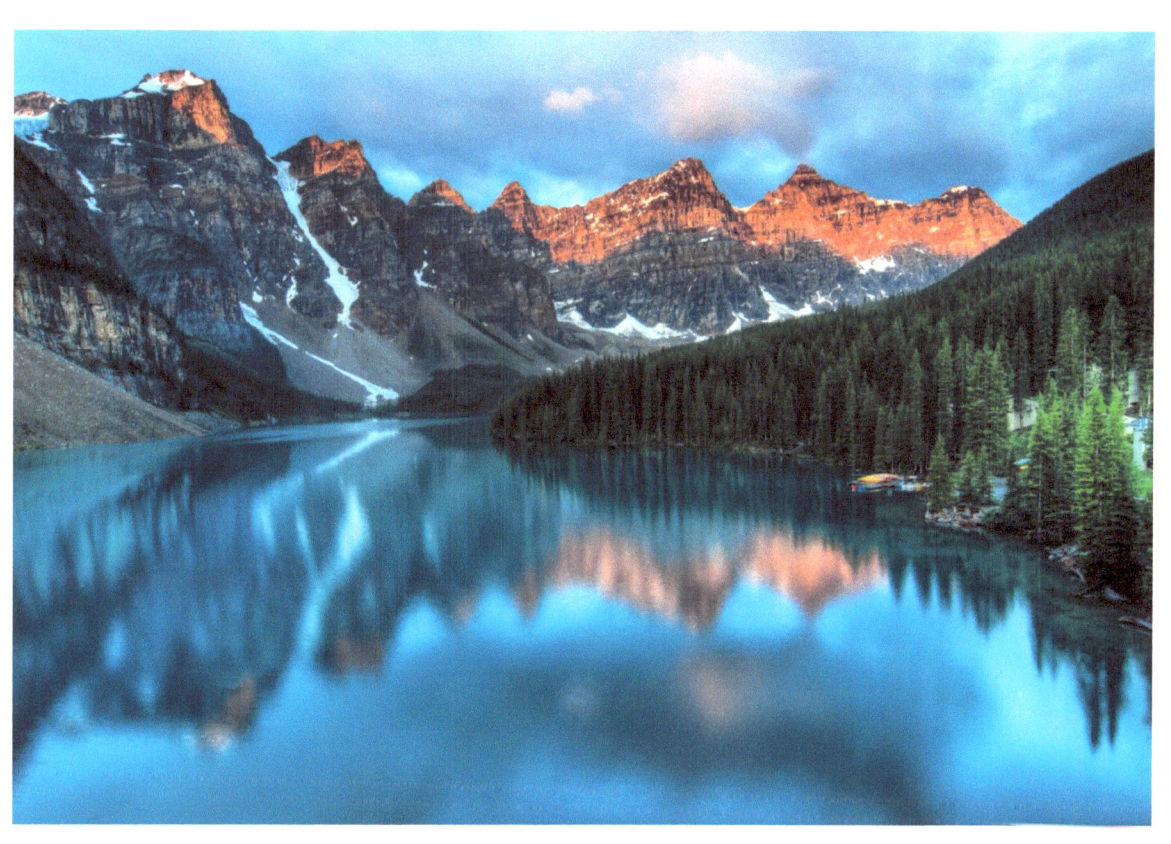

Copyright © 2023 by Hassan Kattan

All rights reserved.

No portion of this book may be reproduced in any form without written permission from the publisher or author, except as permitted by U.S. copyright law.

www.ingramcontent.com/pod-product-compliance
Lightning Source LLC
Chambersburg PA
CBHW051835210526
45473CB00005B/1889